Vegan Diet

14-Day Ketogenic Meal Plan Suitable for Vegans

(Above 50 Vegan Recipes for Permanent Weight Loss, to Manage Body Fat and Stay Fit)

Luis Crump

Published by Robert Satterfield Publishing House

Vegan Diet: 14-Day Ketogenic Meal Plan Suitable for Vegans (Above 50 Vegan Recipes for Permanent Weight Loss, to Manage Body Fat and Stay Fit)

ISBN 978-1-989787-05-2

Legal & Disclaimer

The information contained in this book is not designed to replace or take the place of any form of medicine or professional medical advice. The information in this book has been provided for educational and entertainment purposes only.

The information contained in this book has been compiled from sources deemed reliable, and it is accurate to the best of the Author's knowledge; however, the Author cannot guarantee its accuracy and validity and cannot be held liable for any errors or omissions. Changes are periodically made to this book. You must consult your doctor or get professional medical advice before using any of the suggested remedies, techniques, or information in this book.

TABLE OF CONTENT

Part 1

Introduction

There are as many reasons to become vegan, as there are people who become vegan. Before you start this new lifestyle, it is important to make a conscious decision on why you want to become vegan. Taking this simple step can help you stay motivated.

Why you want to be a Vegan

One of the reasons that many people choose to become vegan is to do their personal part in helping to solve world hunger. In the next year, over 20 million people will die of malnutrition. If each American just reduced their intake of meat by 10 percent, over 100 million people could have adequate nutrition. The reason is that livestock eats over 80 percent of corn and 95 percent of the oats grown in the United States. While 40,000 potatoes can be grown on an acre of land, only 250 pounds of beef can be produced on that same acre.

Other people choose to start living the vegan lifestyle because they are concerned about the harmful effects that raising livestock has on the environment. Over 260 million acres of United States forest has been cleared to produce cropland. It is not, however, just a United States problem. As more cattle than ever before is being rose in rainforest. For each cow that is raised, 55 square feet of rainforest must be cleared. Additionally, it takes three times more fossil fuel to produce a meat-centered diet than a meat-free diet.

Others are concerned that the world may run out of water. It takes much less water to grow a plant-based diet than it does a meat-based diet. For example, it takes 5,000 gallons of water to raise a cow in California, but only 25 gallons to raise a pound of wheat. In fact, raising livestock uses more than half of the water used in the world.

Others are very concerned about getting cancer and know that eating vegan can greatly lower the possibilities that they get this dreaded disease. For example, women who eat eggs on a daily basis are 2.8 times more likely to get ovarian cancer than those who never eat an egg. It is not just women. Men who eat a diet high in dairy products and eggs are 3.6 times more likely to get prostate cancer.

Still others fear that they will die of a fatal heart attack. Researchers found that those individuals who ate a meat-centered diet had an average cholesterol level of 210 mg/dl. They also found that those who lived a vegan lifestyle lowered their chance of having a heart attack by 90 percent.

While many people believe that we are just one plane ride away from a really bad virus spreading around the world, the truth is that bad virus is much more likely to enter your home through the meat you consume if you choose to eat meat. The reason is that 55 percent of all livestock in the United States are fed antibiotics. Then, when you get sick, those antibiotics do not work because your body has already become immune to them.

Other people have problems with their conscious when they eat meat. About 660,000 animals are killed in the United States each hour to provide meat for dinner tables. The problem does not stop there. Those working in slaughterhouses have one of the highest incidences of on the job injuries. Some who choose to eat a vegan lifestyle do so because they feel that it allows them to better connect spiritually with the rest of the world. Some even take this a step further; thinking that what they cause to be infected on others they will face in a coming life.

Benefits of Being a Vegan

For many people the major reason to live a vegan lifestyle is that it is healthier way to live. As already mentioned, eating a vegan diet lowers the risk of cancer and lowers cholesterol. Furthermore, eating a vegan diet has been shown to lower the risk of developing adult onset diabetes. In fact, when researchers conducted a study of 40,000 participants, they found that diabetes occurred four times as often in those eating meat than in those who did not eat meat. When those eating a vegan diet were compared to those eating a vegetarian diet, research showed that vegetarians were two times more likely to develop diabetes than those who ate a vegan diet. Furthermore, researchers found these results held true regardless of ethnicity.

Doctors know that being overweight equates to developing many health problems. Those eating a vegan lifestyle are more likely to have a healthy body mass.

Scientists have learned that eating a plant-rich diet also helps to protect against hypothyroidism. When respondents are further tested, those eating a vegan lifestyle are even more likely not to develop hypothyroidism than those who eat a vegetarian lifestyle.

While it is very easy to understand that eating a diet high in fruits and vegetables is better for the heart, lowers the risk of hypothyroidism, and lowers the risk of diabetes, it surprises many people to know that people who live the vegan lifestyle have fewer eye problems. In fact, doctors have found that people who eat a vegan diet have far fewer cataracts.

The vitamins, minerals and phytochemicals found in the vegan diet also helps to control inflammation in the body. Doctors have found that eating a vegan diet lowers the risk of rheumatoid arthritis, especially when gluten is also eliminated from the diet.

Eating a vegan diet promotes a healthier phosphate level in the body. Therefore, people eating this diet have fewer chronic kidney problems.

If you find the thought of living forever to be attractive, then make sure to consider the vegan lifestyle. Those individuals who carefully monitor their nutrient needs have been shown to enjoy a much longer life. What is even more exciting, they tend to enjoy better health, so that they can enjoy the years they have been blessed to live.

Hurdles to Overcome

There are many reasons that you may want to start living a vegan lifestyle, yet many people consider it difficult to live that lifestyle. Therefore, it is essential to overcome hurdles that you will find stand in your way.

A major hurdle for some people is that they set unrealistic expectations. While most people find that their health improves when they start living a vegan lifestyle, it will not cure everyone's problems. Therefore, it is necessary to have realistic expectations of what the lifestyle will do for you.

Some people who start to live the vegan lifestyle find it hard to control the nutrients in their diets. In particular, they have trouble getting enough B12, Vitamin D, and DHA. Not getting enough of these nutrients in the diet can lead to depression, affect concentration levels, cause fatigue and cause vague aches and pains. Therefore, it is essential either take supplements or eat foods fortified with these nutrients.

People must also carefully control the amount of protein in their diets. The answer to this is to make sure that legumes are regularly consumed as part of the diet. In fact, it is vital to eat at least two servings of legumes every day and some people, especially older adults, find that they need to eat three servings.

There is no doubt about it. The normal vegan diet is lower in fact than either the vegetarian diet or a meat based diet. This often leaves people feeling unsatisfied with their diet. Luckily the answer here is very simple. Just make sure to eat a little bit of healthy fat with every meal.

Some people who begin eating a vegan diet develop anemia or have a low iron rate when their blood is tested. Again, there is an easy solution. Make sure to eat whole grains on a daily basis along with legumes. When eating these foods try combining them with a food that is high in Vitamin C because this vitamin helps the body use the iron found in other foods effectively.

Others who begin this diet find that they have blood sugar spikes. Again, thankfully, there is an easy way to solve this problem. Make sure to eat a diet that is rich in slow carbohydrates like sweet potatoes, oats, barley, quinoa and beans.

Scientists believe that our taste buds are conditioned very early on. If a person has been conditioned to eat animal fat, then they may be conditioned to really like umami. In order to overcome this hurdle, make sure to cook with foods that will bring out umami. Some foods that bring out umami include sundried tomatoes, dried mushrooms, tamari, ripe tomatoes, nutritional yeast, marmite, and sea vegetables. It also matters how you cook your food, because caramelizing, roasting, and grilling produces more umami in foods.

Some people find that cooking vegan begins to control their time. If you start to feel that way, then make sure to look at ways that you can add convenience to your cooking. For example, consider the many vegetarian meat choices found in the freezer section, along with ready-to-use vegetarian cheese options.

Many report feeling isolated, especially when they are first starting to live the vegan lifestyle. There is no need to feel this isolation, as there are many places online where you can find support. After you have become more familiar with the lifestyle, then do not forget to pass your new knowledge on to others.

There are many reasons to embrace the vegan lifestyle. For some, it is the chance to make the world a better place, while for others it is a chance to improve their own health. Scientists know that eating a diet high in plants and eliminating meat and meat products from the diet is a great way to improve many health conditions including lowering cholesterol, stopping cancer, and maintaining a healthy body weight. Not everyone finds it easy to start and maintain a vegan lifestyle. Therefore, it is best to find someone who is already on the diet to mentor you along the way. While we have looked at some of the common nutrient concerns that you will want to keep in mind, the next chapters will examine the diet more closely.

I am very happy to share with you this e-book normally priced at $7.95 for a limited time FREE with your purchase of the Vegan Diet book, I am sure it will help you enormously to achieve your goals and become healthier.

The link to download this fantastic e-book is at the end of this book. Or you can click on the image bellow to take you directly there.

Chapter 1 -Why Home-Cooked Meals are Healthier and Cheaper

Many people who start living a vegan lifestyle find that it is much easier to prepare the majority of their meals at home. Instead of considering this a burden, there are many reasons that it is healthier and cheaper to prepare meals at home.

The budget conscious consumer finds that they can save lots of money by preparing meals at home. In fact, author Laura Stec proves that it is easy to save over $100 just by taking meals to work. Making it even better to prepare meals at home, food can often be bought in bulk and cooked in many different ways and saving money by using store coupons. Making it even easier, many vegan meals are perfect for freezing.

Many people do not take into consideration the total amount of time that it takes to eat in a restaurant. First, if you have a family, you must take the time to round everyone up. Often an argument pursues about where to eat and the winning restaurant always seems to be clear across town through impossible traffic. Even if you live by yourself, you must drive to the restaurant, wait to be seated, and then wait for the server to take your order. Then, comes the longest wait of all, as you wait for someone to prepare your food. If you are like many people, you then rush through the meal, because you need to be somewhere else. Finally, you have to drive home. Eliminating all those hassles is easy when you cook at home. Making it even easier, if you know that you are going to be busy on a particular night, planning for leftovers or cooking ahead is easy.

It is hard to find vegan options in many restaurants. Even if you take the time to read the menu carefully and talk to the server, there are still no guarantees. Additionally, foods prepared in restaurants are usually higher in trans-fats and salt. When you prepare meals at home, it is easy to control what is in your food, how much fat and salt you are eating and prepare the foods according to your own taste buds.

In order to stay healthy, a variety of different options need to be included in the diet. It is much easier to provide balanced meals when you cook at home. That way, you can make sure that you are getting enough protein, Vitamin D, Vitamin B12 and other essential nutrients in your diet in the right amounts.

Over 76 million Americans are poisoned by the food that they eat each year. When you prepare foods at home, it is easy to make sure that everything is spotless before you begin cooking. It is also easy to make sure that you are preparing foods to the right temperatures and storing foods properly.

When you eat right, you have enough energy to last throughout even the most trying day. After all, everyone seems to be running from the time the alarm goes off in the morning until long after the time a person should go to bed. When an individual cooks at home t is easy to add some extra fruit as a natural pick me up, but almost impossible, when one eats out, as these choices are usually extremely limited and very expensive.

Research out of the University of Michigan shows that it is vital for young people to eat at home. They show that families who regularly eat with their families enjoy higher academic success and less delinquency problems. After all, we are what we eat, so cooking at home allows people to determine what their children will become. It is also very easy for people to incorporate everyone into the cooking process so that parents can pass on important ideas about the food that they eat and the knowledge about how to prepare those foods to their children. Since very few people choose to eat vegan, it is important to pass on this skillset and cooking techniques early before children are allowed to go places on their own.

Most restaurants are serving larger portions than ever before. In fact, a study published in the Journal of Public Health Policy showed that the average dinner plate used in a restaurant went up two inches in size between 1990 and 2010. This encourages people to eat more food than ever before when dining out. While dining at home allows people to more easily control their portion sizes. The result is that people eat much less food allowing people to more easily control their weight.

Home cooked meals are healthier and cheaper than eating out for so many different reasons. It is very easy to control what you are putting in your body when you eat at home. Not only can you control the types of food that you are eating, but also the amount of food, so that everyone gets exactly what they need. You really are what you eat, so you should be in control of this aspect of your life, as opposed to a chef in a restaurant.

Chapter 2 -Define What's Vegan

The simple definition of what's vegan is that it is any food that does not come from an animal in any way. Therefore, not only do people on a vegan diet not choose to eat meat, but they also avoid dairy products that come from animals. The vegan diet is one of the most demanding diets to follow, so it is important to take it beyond the basic definition.

In order to make sure that a person is eating a balanced vegan diet, think about a pyramid. Whole grains form the base of the vegan diet and are essential for energy. The vegan dieter needs to make sure that they are consuming complex carbohydrates to make sure that they have the energy to keep going all day. There are many foods that fall within the grain group including quinoa, barley, corn, millet, barley and barley. Many people following this diet eat whole grain breads and start the day with a big bowl of grain.

The next level of the pyramid consists of fruits and vegetables. In order to keep the diet balanced without spending hours trying to balance different nutrients on paper, try to consume many different colors of fruits and vegetables each day. Luckily, the dieter finds so many different choices:

Red- red potatoes, strawberries, red apples, beets

Blue- blueberries, blue potatoes, blue lettuce

Green- green grapes, greens, asparagus, broccoli, avocadoes

Purple- purple grapes, plums, blackberries

Orange- sweet potatoes, pumpkins, carrots, cantaloupes

Yellow- squash, mangos, bananas, yellow apples

While many people will find a variety of choices at local grocery stores, do not overlook the possibility of finding unique options at local farmer's markets. In particular, try to find one where heirloom fruits and vegetables are sold or consider growing your own.

Setting on top of the fruits and vegetable level are the legumes. It is not only important that you eat at least four servings from this group each day, but also that you eat a variety of different legumes. Thankfully, there are many different options, including split peas, kidney beans, cannellini beans, lentils, chickpeas, and split peas.

Many people grew up in a household where drinking milk was considered an absolute necessity. That is simply not the case. After all, humans are the only primates that drink milk after they mature. Yet, people still need many of the nutrients that come from the milk group. That is why it is necessary to get two to four servings from the milk group each day. Thankfully, there are many great options including almond milk, hemp milk, hazelnut milk, soymilk, and rice milk. Not only are these great options for drinking, but also many work very well when baking.

At the top of the vegan food pyramid are fats and oils. While many people have been taught that this group should be avoided, that is simply not the case. It is vital, however, that this group be eaten in moderation. Without any fat in the diet, people are not satisfied with their diets, because it encourages a person to feel full. Fats also are essential for many body functions to perform properly. There are many great options including olive oil and coconut oil. Not all fat needs to come in the form of cooking oil, however, as there are many fruits and vegetables that contain some fat such as avocadoes and olives. Additionally, do not forget about nuts and seeds as a way to put healthy fats into your diet.

Vegan Ingredients-Where to Find Them

People who are just starting on a vegan diet often worry about where they will get the ingredients that they need to cook their meals. The great news is that the local grocery stores are usually loaded with wonderful options that work. The key is to make sure to read package ingredient list to make sure that they do not contain ingredients that you do not want, because they tend to sneak in places that you would never suspect.

Remember that it is not always necessary to start out with individual ingredients to enjoy success on the vegan diet. For example, many boxed cereals and prepackaged porridges contain only allowed ingredients. The careful shopper finds many whole grain pastas along with whole grain baking mixes. In the frozen food section, shoppers find frozen whole grain pancakes, waffles, pizza crusts, tortillas and frozen breads. Meanwhile, shopping the bread aisle yields whole grain loaves, pita bread, bagels, English muffins, rolls and baguettes. Many of these same choices are available in the bakery section of larger grocery stores.

The dieter will also find many choices when it comes to buying legumes. Many different varieties of legumes can usually be found including mung, soybeans, Northern, lima, chickpeas, black-eyed peas and navy. Do not stop with shopping just this one aisle, however, as shoppers can find tofu, and lentil burgers on other aisles in the store.

Nuts are a wonderful addition to the vegan diet. Packages can be found in the grocery store, but do not overlook the savings when buying in bulk. Bulk nuts are often located in or near the produce section at grocery stores.

Fresh fruits and vegetables are found in the produce section, but do not stop shopping there, as the frozen section is a great place to find foods that may not currently be in season.

While a trip to the grocery store is a great place to get ingredients for your vegan diet experience, do not overlook shopping at local farmer's markets. The advantage of shopping at these markets is that often fruits and vegetables can be found that are missing in most grocery stores. The reason is that the vendors can usually afford to grow their products in smaller amounts allowing them to offer a greater variety. You may find that many vendors offer heirloom fruits and vegetables that are great additions to your diet, as they often offer different nutrients than found in the grocery store choices. Incorporating these choices also is an outstanding way to introduce greater variety in your diet so that you do not get bored of eating the same old thing.

Another option that many people eating the vegan diet enjoy is growing their own foods. Even people that live in apartment complexes can enjoy growing food in pots in their apartments. Additionally, many apartment communities enjoy square foot gardening. Finally, do not overlook the possibility of community gardens in your area. If you do not find one, then think about organizing one yourself.

Finding the ingredients for a vegan diet is not difficult. Foods can be found at the local grocery store, and it is not always necessary to start from scratch with all foods. The local farmer's market is another great source that may offer even more variety. Additionally, many people endorse raising their own food when eating the vegan lifestyle.

Chapter 3 -Prepare Your Kitchen to Cook

Easy and Quick

Embracing the vegan lifestyle starts with preparing your kitchen. Start by removing all ingredients that do not fit with your new lifestyle. If you cannot stand to throw things away, then donate them to a worthwhile cause, as you will enjoy the benefits of knowing that you have helped someone else. Not having these items in your home also means that you will not be tempted to return to your former lifestyle.

Make sure that everything is spotless. Most foodborne illnesses happen when food is not prepared in a clean environment. Since you are likely to spend more time cooking at home than in recent days, if the budget allows, now may be the perfect time to update your kitchen. Even a fresh coat of paint can signal that you are embracing a new way to live.

Make sure that your kitchen has plenty of space to gather. If you are a parent, then consider creating special counters that are low enough for children to easily work as they will love to help. Additionally, if you are a music lover or a television addict, think about how you can incorporate these items into your kitchen. If you enjoy a glass of wine while cooking, then incorporate these areas too.

Tools

While you can start the vegan lifestyle with what you currently have on hand when it comes to tools that you already have on hand, you will find that having certain utensils makes your life much easier.

The first of these tools is a food steamer. There are two basic types of food steamers. One sits on the countertop and all the user needs to do is put the food in and set the timer, as the steamer does the work itself. Designed to sit on the stovetop, the second type is a pot that the user fills with water and then inserts a basket with vegetables at the top. It is important, however, to realize that a stovetop steamer needs to be carefully monitored, so that it does not boil dry.

The advantage of the second type of steamer is that they usually cost a lot less than an electric steamer, so if money is tight, it is definitely the way to go. When looking at stovetop steamers, the cheapest option is the stainless steel version. While they work very well in many cases, most do not adjust very well to different sizes of pans so you may need more than one. These also get very hot so the cook needs to use them with care.

Another option for stovetop steamers is the silicone option. One major advantage here is that they do not get hot. Therefore, the novice cook often finds them easier to work with in the kitchen. Many come with large handles that make them even easier to handle. Since they are soft, they will not scratch pots causing coatings to come off in the food.

Most people who endorse the vegan lifestyle, however, will want to invest in an electric steamer. The best electric steamers have multiple layers allowing many different foods to be cooked at the same time.

If you are considering an electric steamer, then consider ones that allow you to do multiple things. For example, some units allow you to steam, pressure cook, and slow cook which can be a huge space saving convenience. When looking at these units, look for ones that are made of stainless steel as they will stand up longer and eliminate the harmful effects of plastic on the body.

The second tool that the vegan cook will need is a pressure cooker since they allow for fast meal preparation. As we have already covered, it is possible to find a steamer, pressure cooker and slow cooker as one unit. Having a separate non-electric pressure cooker is an option that many people will want to consider because they can be used on gas stove tops if the electricity goes out. Some models are designed to be used on campfires for those who enjoy an active lifestyle.

The third tool that almost every vegan cook needs is a good blender, as they are useful for so many different purposes, such as making soups and smoothies. When shopping for a blender, consider those with attachments that allow you to do many different things. Additionally, blenders come with different size motors. The larger the motor, the more powerful the machine will be. Therefore, it will handle harder fruits and vegetables easier.

The cook also needs a variety of pots and pans. One thing that the cook needs to consider when buying pots and pans, is to find some where food will not stick. This is particularly important when preparing high-protein foods, such as tofu, are notorious for sticking. Not all non-stick pans are created equal, and many people are aware that Teflon has been shown to possibly cause cancer when it flakes off into food. Therefore, look for options where the pan is constructed of a non-stick material so you do not need to worry about the coating flaking off.

Generally, the heavier the pan, the longer it will last. While these pans can be more expensive to begin with, they often last longer allowing the buyer to save money in the long run. One popular option encases a layer of aluminum between two stainless steel options allowing the pan to heat evenly.

The cook needs a variety of pan sizes, as it is important to never overcrowd the food in a pan because it stops the food from cooking evenly. The heavier the layer of aluminum, the more likely the pan is to heat evenly.

While plastic containers are still a popular option for storing many food options, it may not be the best choice. The truth is that researchers still do not fully understand what impact using plastic is having on harmful chemicals leeching into food. Therefore, the cook should consider using glass instead.

There are also several smaller tools that a person preparing a vegan diet will need. The first of these is several good chef knives. All knives should have ergonomically designed handles, so that the individual can use them easily. The blade should extend inside the handle as this provides added strength.

There is debate as to rather a ceramic knife or a stainless steel knife is better. Those who prefer stainless steel knives point out the ease that these knives can be sharpened when necessary, while the others point out that ceramic knives stay sharper longer and generally last longer.

You will also need a variety of other tools in your kitchen that you may already have on hand. Alternatively, you may want to celebrate your new lifestyle by getting new ones. Some of the most important ones will be a salad spinner, grater, garlic press, whisks, measuring spoons, measuring cups, tongs, colanders, and strainers. One very useful tool that you will want to get is a small coffee grinder, as it is very useful for grinding seeds into powder for including n your spice blends and tossing on your salads.

Spices

One area that many people complain about when starting to eat the vegan diet is that the diet is bland. By themselves, many foods on the vegan diet have milder flavors, but those foods are great for enhancing with herbs and spices. If you have not priced these ingredients lately, buying them all at once can greatly add to your grocery bill. There are several tips that you can use to save money when buying spices.

Each person has their own flavors that they love. These are the spices that a person needs to buy in bulk. Other spices that you need for an occasional dish should be purchased in the smallest amount possible. Many people find it helpful to buy all their spices in containers to begin with, but then find places that will sell these herbs and spices and refill the bottles.

Never overlook the possibility of growing herbs at home. While this can be easily accomplished, you will want to keep your pantry stocked with some basic herbs such as bay leaves, dill, basil, thyme, oregano, dill, rosemary, garlic powder, nutmeg, turmeric, ground cinnamon, nutmeg, ground ginger, paprika, onion powder and chili powder.

You will discover that you are using more pepper than ever before. A great way to make sure that you are using the freshest possible pepper is to buy black peppercorns and a peppermill. When purchasing a peppermill, look for one where you can easily adjust the grind based on what you are cooking. While you may find that you want to limit the amount of salt in your cooking, having a variety of salts on hand ensures such as

Himalayan salt, sea salt, and kosher salt allows you to use salt creatively.

Stock up on the ethnic spices based on the cuisine that you like to eat the best. If you love Italian cuisine, then stock up on red pepper flakes and fennel. Alternatively, if you love Asian cuisine, then consider coriander, star anise, cardamom, curry powder, cumin, and garmam masalala and five-spice powder. If you prefer Tex-Mex and Spanish cuisine, then make sure to stock up on cumin, coriander chili powder, cayenne pepper, and Mexican oregano. It is usually cheaper to buy individual spices and create your own blends. If you do not know what is in a certain blend, then check the Internet because you will find many suggestions.

You may discover that you love to bake now that you are starting your vegan lifestyle. If this is true, then you will certainly want to stock up on baking spices such as ginger, cloves, cream of tartar, nutmeg, and cinnamon.

While you are buying your spices, it is important to think about how you plan to store them. While many spices come in plastic jars, it is better to store spices in glass jars. Spices will last longer when stored between 40 and 70 degrees and keep them away from light. Most spices will keep six months and many will keep much longer. If the flavor begins to change, then it is time to discard it, and buy some new. Likewise, if you examine your spices carefully, most will change colors just before they begin to go bad. Some spices are high in natural oils and they can become rancid.

Your kitchen should become a place that you enjoy spending your time. Therefore, consider ways that you can upgrade it so that you can enjoy it even more. Even if major renovations are not in the budget right now, then think about a place that people can gather and give the room a fresh coat of paint. Get the tools and gadgets that will make your life easier, such as a steamer and a pressure cooker.

Finally, eliminate the ho-hums when it comes to eating this new diet by getting a wide variety of spices.

Chapter 4 -5 Vegan Recipes for Breakfast

Many people who are not familiar with the vegan diet think that breakfast may be a tough meal to prepare on this diet, because they limit there thinking to salads and vegetable soups. In fact, there are many vegan breakfast options that you will adore. Here are five vegan recipes for breakfast that will help you start your day right.

Skillet Scramble

Ingredients

4 small red potatoes

1/2 medium yellow onion

1/2 red bell pepper

1 small bunch Swiss chard

2 tablespoons olive oil, divided

6 ounces vegan sausage

1 pound extra-firm tofu, drained, pressed, and cut into 1/2-inch dice

2 cloves garlic

1 cup sliced cremini mushrooms

1 teaspoon dried basil

1 teaspoon dried parsley

1 teaspoon dried thyme

1 teaspoon salt

1/2 teaspoon turmeric

1/8 teaspoon cayenne pepper

2 tablespoons lemon juice

3 tablespoons nutritional yeast

Instructions

1.Peel potatoes and slice into one-inch cubes. Place them in a steamer and steam for about 14 minutes until tender.

2. Meanwhile, coarsely chop the pepper and onion.

3. Remove the stems from the Swiss chard and tear into bite size pieces.

4. After the potatoes have been steamed, place the oil into a skillet. Lightly brown

the potatoes and set them aside on a plate.

5. Add the onion to the skillet and cook for about two minutes.

6. Crumble the sausage into the skillet and cook for two more minutes.

7. Drain and press the tofu and cut into small pieces. Add it to the sausage and onions.

8. Add the chard and mushrooms. Cook for 15 minutes until the tofu begins to turn a gold color.

9. Add the basil, parsley, thyme, salt, turmeric, cayenne pepper, and nutritional yeast.

10. Return the potatoes to the skillet.

11. Add the lemon juice and cook for about five minutes until everything is warm.

Banana Muffins

1/4 cup unsweetened applesauce

1/4 cup non-dairy butter

1 cup organic granulated sugar

2 teaspoons organic soy flour

2 Tablespoons water

2 bananas

1 cup whole wheat flour

1 cup unbleached flour

1 teaspoon baking powder

1/2 teaspoon baking soda

1 cup non-dairy milk

1 tablespoon apple cider vinegar

1 teaspoon vanilla extract

Instructions:

1.Preheat oven to 375 degrees.

2. Lightly grease a muffin pan.

3. Place the applesauce, non-dairy spread, sweetener in a mixing bowl and cream until well combined.

4. In a small bowl, combine the soy flour and water. Then, fold the mixture into the applesauce mixture.

5. Mash the bananas and fold them into the mixture.

6. Add the vanilla. Then, slowly add the whole-wheat flour, unbleached flour, baking soda and baking powder.

7. Combine the non-dairy milk and apple cider vinegar in a bowl. Then, add to the mixture.

8. After ensuring that everything is well combined, pour the batter into the muffin cups so that each cup is 3/4 full.

9. Bake for 24 minutes until a toothpick inserted in the middle of the muffin comes out clean.

10. Immediately remove the muffins to a wire rack and allow cooling.

Pumpkin Oatmeal

Ingredients

1/3-cup regular oats

1-cup non-dairy milk

1/2-teaspoon vanilla extract

1/2-cup pumpkin

1/2-tablespoon chia seeds

1/8-teaspoon sea salt

1/2-teaspoon cinnamon

1/4-teaspoon ginger

1/8-teaspoon nutmeg

1 tablespoon chopped pecans

1 tablespoon almond milk

1-tablespoon maple syrup

1/2 teaspoon Earth Balance

1/3 Pumpkin Butter Oat Square

Instructions

1.Heat oats and almond milk to a slow boil over medium heat.

2. Stir in pumpkin and chia seeds. Continue cooking for six minutes stirring frequently.

3. Stir in the sea salt, cinnamon, ginger, nutmeg and vanilla extract. Cook another

five minutes stirring frequently. Remove from the heat.

4. Crumble the pumpkin butter oat square into a small bowl. Add the Earth Balance, maple syrup, almond milk and pecans.

5. Place the oatmeal mixture into a bowl and top with the pumpkin butter oat square mixture.

.

Blueberry Muffins

1-cup non-dairy milk

1-tablespoon apple cider vinegar

1/4-cup ground flax seed

1-cup whole wheat

3/4 cup all-purpose flour)

1 1/2 teaspoon baking soda

1-teaspoon ground cinnamon

1/4-teaspoon kosher salt

1/4-cup olive oil

1/2-cup pure maple syrup

1-teaspoon vanilla extract

1/2 teaspoon almond extract

1 1/2 cup blueberries

2 1/2 tablespoons organic granulated sugar

1-teaspoon cinnamon

2 teaspoons Earth Balance

2 teaspoons flour

1/8-teaspoon salt

Instructions

1.Preheat oven to 375 degrees. Line a 24-hole mini muffin tin with liners.

2. In a medium-mixing bowl, combine the ground flax, flour, baking soda, cinnamon and salt.

3. In a small bowl, combine the non-dairy milk and the apple cider vinegar.

4. After five minutes, add the oil, syrup, vanilla and almond extract to the non-dairy milk.

5. Add the wet ingredients to the dry ingredients stirring until just combined.

6. Spoon the mixture into the paper liners.

7. Combine the remaining ingredients and gently sprinkle on the top.

8. Bake for about 17 minutes until the top of the muffins spring back when lightly touched.

9. Tip the muffins on their edges as soon as you take them out of the oven.

10. As soon as possible, remove the muffins from the pan and allow to cool on a wire rack.

8 cups Italian bread cubes

6 ounces silken tofu

1/2 cup packed light brown sugar

2 teaspoons vanilla extract

1-teaspoon ground cinnamon

1/4-teaspoon ground nutmeg

1/8-teaspoon allspice

1/4 teaspoon. salt

2 cups plain unsweetened nondairy milk

1/4-cup pure maple syrup, plus more for serving

1-tablespoon vegan butter

1/4 cup coarsely chopped pecans

Ingredients

1.Preheat the oven to 275 degrees.

2. Cut the bread not bite size pieces and place them on a baking sheet.

3. Spread the bread on a baking sheet. Place it in the oven for 30 minutes.

4. Spray the inside of a slow cooker generously with cooking spray.

5. Transfer the dry breadcrumbs to the slow cooker.

6. Combine the sugar, tofu, vanilla, cinnamon, nutmeg, salt and all spice in a food processor.

7. Add the maple syrup and milk blending until just combined.

8. Pour the mixture over the bread.

9. Dot with vegan butter and top with pecans.

10. Cook on high until firm that will take about one hour.

Chapter 5 -5 Vegan Recipes for Lunch

Mexican Tempeh Quinoa Salad

Ingredients

1-cup quinoa

2 cups water

1-tablespoon olive oil

1/2 onion

1 red pepper

8 ounces tempeh

1-cup salsa

1-tablespoon lime juice

1-teaspoon cumin

1/4-teaspoon cayenne pepper

1/4-teaspoon salt

1/4-teaspoon pepper

15 ounces black beans

1-cup fresh corn

1/2-cup cherry tomatoes

2 tablespoons fresh cilantro

1/8-teaspoon salt

1/8-teaspoon pepper

1 avocado

Directions

1.Pour the quinoa and water into a Dutch oven with a tight fitting lid. Bring to a boil, then reduce heat and let it simmer 20 minutes covered. Once all the water is absorbed, fluff it with a fork.

2. Meanwhile, dice the pepper and onion. Once the quinoa is cooked, add them to the pan

3. Cut the tempeh into bite size pieces and add it to the pan

4. Add the seasonings, the lime juice and the salsa. Cook over low heat stirring frequently for 15 minutes

5. Transfer the mixture to a glass bowl

6. Drain and rinse the black beans and add them to the mixture

7. Dice the tomato and cilantro and add them to the pan. Add the corn, salt and pepper. Stir until well combined

8. Dice the avocado and stir it in

Sweet Potato Salad

Ingredients

4 large sweet potatoes

1/2-cup extra-virgin olive oil

1/8-teaspoon salt

1/8 teaspoon coarsely ground black pepper

1/4-cup red-wine vinegar

1 medium red bell pepper

2 teaspoons ground cumin

1 tablespoon grated orange zest

1/2 cup sliced scallion

1/2 cup minced fresh mint leaves

1 jalapeño

1/4-cup raisins

Directions

1.Preheat the oven to 400°

2. Peel the sweet potatoes and cut into bite-sized pieces

3. Place the pieces on a baking sheet and drizzle six tablespoons of the oil over the potatoes and toss to coat

4. Season the potatoes with the salt and pepper

5. Put the potatoes in the oven and roast for 15 minutes

6. Remove the baking sheet from the oven and flip the potatoes over. Return the potatoes to the oven for another 15 minutes

7. Meanwhile, in a blender, combine the remaining oil, vinegar, orange zest, and cumin

8. Dice the bell pepper and add it to the mixture. Puree until smooth

9. Toss the warm potatoes with the remaining ingredients. Then add the dressing a little at a time. Depending on your taste buds, you may not need all the dressing

Quinoa and Cumin-Spiced Lentils

Ingredients

6 carrots

6 stalks celery

1 white onion

1 tomato

1 cup dried quinoa

 2 cups organic vegetable broth

15 ounces can black beans

1/8-teaspoon salt

1/8-teaspoon pepper

1-tablespoon olive oil

8 ounces dried green lentils

1-quart vegetable broth

1/4-teaspoon ground coriander

1/4-teaspoon ground cumin

1/8-teaspoon salt

1/8-teaspoon pepper

Instructions

1. Dice two carrots and slice the remainder

2. Dice the tomatoes and onion

3. Slice the celery into bite sized pieces

4. Sauté the onions in the olive oil until translucent. Add the tomatoes, celery, sliced carrots, spices, vegetable broth, lentils and spices. Cover and cook for one hour over medium heat

5. After the lentil mixture has cooked for about 30 minutes, put the quinoa and organic vegetable broth in a large pot. Bring to a boil

6. Reduce heat and simmer quinoa for 10 minutes

7. Drain and rinse the black beans. Stir them into the quinoa

8. Cook for 17 minutes, then fluff with a fork

9. Spoon the quinoa-bean mixture into six individual serving bowls. Top with the lentil mixture, and enjoy

Summer Delight Curry

Ingredients

1/2 yellow onion

 1 sweet potato

1-inch ginger

2 zucchini

1-tablespoon coconut oil

 2 cloves garlic

1-tablespoon curry powder

1-teaspoon coriander seeds

1-teaspoon cumin seeds

1/2-teaspoon fenugreek seeds

1/2-teaspoon turmeric powder

1 28 ounces canned crushed tomato

14 ounce canned chickpeas

1/2-teaspoon agave nectar

1/2-cup cilantro

1-tablespoon lime juice

Instructions

1.Chop the cilantro, sweet potato and zucchini. Dice the onion. Grate the ginger

2. Heat the coconut oil in a large pan over medium heat. Once hot, add the onion and sweet potato. Cook until the onion is almost translucent

2. Mince the garlic and add it to the onion

3. Add the curry powder, coriander seeds, cumin seeds, fenugreek seeds, and turmeric powder. Cook for one minute

4. Add the crushed tomatoes and bring to a boil

5. Reduce the heat and cover the pan. Simmer for 10 minutes

6. Add the agave nectar, chickpeas, and zucchini. Return the cover to the pan and cook for 11 minutes. If the mixture looks dry, then add a little water

7. Remove from the heat and stir in the cilantro and lime. Serve and enjoy

Slow Cooker Pumpkin Chili

Ingredients

3-pound pie pumpkin

2 medium turnips

½-cup unsalted non-dairy butter

½-cup olive oil

½-cup cornmeal

2 red bell peppers

1 large onion

6 garlic cloves

2 tablespoons tomato paste

4 cups organic vegetarian broth

20 ounce canned diced tomatoes with green chilies

32 ounce cans chili beans

2 cups frozen corn

1-tablespoon chili powder

1-teaspoon cinnamon

1-teaspoon cumin

1/8-teaspoon salt

1/8-teaspoon pepper

1-tablespoon balsamic vinegar,

Instructions

1.Cut the pumpkin in half and take out the seeds and strings

2. Place each half, cut side down, in a shallow pan of water and microwave for five minutes

3. Let the pumpkin cool. Use a sharp knife to remove the skin

4. Peel the turnips and cube into bite size pieces

5. In a soup pot, heat the non-dairy butter and olive oil over medium heat.

6. Stir in the cornmeal

7. Cut the peeled pumpkin into bite sized pieces and add it to the turnips

8. Chop the bell pepper and onion and add them

9. Mince the garlic and add it

10. Add the tomato paste and cook 10 minutes

11. Add the remaining ingredients and bring to a boil

12 Reduce the heat and simmer for one hour

Conclusion

To be a Vegan can prove difficult, especially if you are a very social person and like to go out with friends. However it's very important o understand why are we consciously deciding to become a vegan. Maybe it's for humanitarian causes, ecological, healthy or other causes. But it should always be an important deeply personal reason on why we are deciding to skip de food many people eat on their every day diet.

If you have this reasons clear and you feel at heart that you are doing the correct thing, it will be very easy to follow the different concepts of a Vegan diet, even more important you will start to feel great and enjoy greatly the benefits eating Vegan.

Your body will be healthier and you will feel lighter and have more energy. You will feel you can focus your mind better and even lose weight.

However it's very important to understand that although in this book I gave you a very good introduction on how to become a vegan, you should always discuss it with an expert in the nutritional field on how you can balance your food intake for your specific personal needs so you always eat a balanced amount of the different nutrients that your body needs.

If you follow the steps and decide to embrace the Vegan lifestyle I wish you all the luck and enjoy a healthy and delicious lifestyle.

Part 2

Chapter 1 - Introduction

In the modern day scenario, with our hectic schedules and unhealthy lifestyles, we are often gripped by innumerable ailments and some of them are really fatal and cause great damage in the long run. At the end of a long and tiring day, we are too tired to fix up a healthy meal, so we often opt for restaurant meals that come for a price and also go in for processed and fast foods. These food choices might seem like heaven and very comforting when you are consuming it, but overtime, it can lead to immense weight gain and also lead to lots of modern day ailments, including, obesity, diabetes, blood pressure, depression and anxiety among several other complications.

Most of us are busy chasing our professional goals that we often compromise on our health and fitness. Sedentary lifestyle is the root cause for most of the damage done in terms of health. Sedentary lifestyle can cause great harm to health and also lead one to develop low self-esteem and loss of confidence when he or she realizes that they have lost much in the quest of making a career and money. Needless to say, health is an integral part of life and without health everything else is a lost cause. If you have been neglecting this essential part of life, then it is time to wake up, take notice and act to save the day. If this situation sounds similar then this is the guide that you need to snap out of your unhealthy way of life and start afresh.

If you wish to adopt a healthy lifestyle that offers much energy, good health and well-being, then try life the vegan way as explained in this guide. Besides ensuring an energetic and fit body, it also leads to effective weight loss. The best part about adopting a vegan lifestyle is that it does not let you compromise with your health at any cost. It provides all the essentials that your body needs, while still ensuring weight loss and immense energy and fitness.

In this guide we will provide extensive information around a vegan diet for beginners. It will also throw light on all aspects of a vegan lifestyle, including its essentials, what it encompasses, why you should go vegan, kitchen essentials, some useful tips, and recipes for a complete vegan meal plan. For all those aiming for weight loss and restoration of energy and good health, this guide will prove handy and useful to attain their cause. Try out the interesting and delicious recipes provided in this guide and you will be glad to live life the vegan way and will be left asking for more, lots more! Read on for some healthy options.

Chapter 2 - What is a Vegan Diet?

Vegan diet is a type of diet which is very similar to a vegetarian diet but it goes much further than just that. A vegan diet shuns the use of anything that is related to animals or processed with the use of animal products. It also boycotts the consumption of meat, dairy products and other ingredients derived from animals and living organisms. All those who follow the vegan style of life are referred to as 'vegans' and the diet itself is referred to as 'veganism'. Some of the ingredients consumed by vegans are as follows:

- They vouch for all varieties of fruits and vegetables as it provides the body with all the essential vitamins and nutrients for a healthy body.
- In addition to that, they also consume a whole variety of starchy foods such as potatoes, rice, grains, bread, pasta, cereals and lots more. It serves as an excellent source of carbohydrates,

which is very crucial for a healthy meal plan.

- Other food options such as beans, legumes, grains, dairy alternatives such as soya, sources of proteins such as pulses and lots more also find place in the diet.
- The diet incorporates a very minute amount of fatty and sugar induced foods but only those which exclude the use of dairy products.
- For all those who wish to deviate a bit but still remain vegan, there are vegan options for almost all goodies like ice creams, cheese, mayonnaise and lots more.

A new vegan follower might fear that his/her daily essentials are not met when they exclude non vegetarian and dairy options from the diet. The good news is that all this can be accounted for even in the vegan way of life.

- Calcium and Vitamin D: foods such as fortified soya, rice, pulses, brown and white bread and even dried fruits such as figs, apricots and raisons, are sufficient to serve the purpose.

- Proteins: protein rich foods such as soya beans, chickpeas, lentils, nuts, seeds, mushrooms, broccoli, whole wheat bread, oatmeal and lots more will do the trick.
- Iron: foods such as pulses, bread, cereals, dark green vegetables like broccoli, spring greens and dried fruits are suitable for a good dose of iron.
- Omega 3 fatty acids: flaxseeds, soya oil, soya rich foods and walnuts are sufficient.
- Calcium: it can easily be gained from broccoli, collard greens, beans, almonds, calcium induced soya or rice milk, orange juice and lots more.

Chapter 3 - Reasons to Select Vegan Diet

The benefits of going vegan are innumerable which vouches for the fact that it is indeed the best approach for a healthy and fit lifestyle. Read on to know more and you will surely gear up to move forth on the path of veganism.

Reduces risk of diseases:

It is definitely the best way to make your body healthier and resistant to several ailments that come as a part and parcel of modern day sedentary lifestyles. It certainly eliminates the risk of several chronic degenerative diseases such as diabetes, obesity, high blood pressure, coronary artery diseases and various types of cancer, such as colon, prostrate, breast, stomach and lung among others.

Aids weight loss:

It is surely the best method to not only lose weight but it also helps you to maintain it once you have got your weight under control. Consuming too many meat and dairy products can lead to an increased accumulation of unhealthy fat and cholesterol in the body. Since this approach only allows healthy food ingredients, it ensures that your body slims down without leading to any deterioration in your health. The elimination of high fat and cholesterol related foods from your diet is a great way to start shedding some of the unwanted weight.

Improves Energy:

It ensures higher levels of energy and boosts your immunity effectively. It also provides your body with all the strength that it requires. It prevents you from feeling fatigued or weak. The consumption of fresh fruits and vegetables acts as bowel regulator and ensures regular movements. This in turn aids the digestive system and leaves you feeling light, active and brisk all day long.

Shuns toxic chemicals:

Most often the products derived from animals such as meat and dairy products are filled with steroids, hormones and other chemical ingredients. They cause great damage to the body and in turn can cause several diseases that attack your body. Sometimes it can even be fatal. Opting for vegetarian options, particularly organic foods, is the safest option.

Saves Our Environment:

According to research, there is a lot of pollution and damage caused by the animal wastes, which is conveniently run into the rivers. It contaminates the drinking water and also leads to many diseases. If you decide to go for the vegan lifestyle, it also vouches for animal rights. You are not torturing them for your eating preferences and you respect their rights to live and grow like every other living creature.

Reduces physical complaints:

Studies show that people who have gone vegan have experienced great difference in their physical health. Apart from increasing the energy levels and flushing out toxins, it also ensures healthy skin and definitely promotes longevity of life. It helps tackle the problem of body odor, bad breathe, migraines, allergies and also keeps PMS symptoms at bay. It is a great way to ensure long tresses and healthy nails and bones.

Chapter 4 - Equipping the Vegan Kitchen

The best part about converting your kitchen into a vegan kitchen is that you do not really require too many types of equipment or shell out big bucks to support the lifestyle change. All you need are some basic tools and you are good to go. Since it is mainly vegetables and fruits, there will be a lot of chopping so make sure you get hold of a chopping board as it makes everything simple and less messy and some great cutting tools. Load up your cutlery with some sharp knives as it greatly simplifies that work to be done. Another great tool is a mandolin, which is like a slicer and very handy for slicing ingredients. However, extreme care should be taken while handling it to prevent any damage to your hands and fingers. Another very useful tool is a garlic press. Garlic acts as an excellent seasoning ingredient and adds great flavor to almost any dish and having a garlic press ready at your disposable is indeed a great idea as it makes mincing and chopping garlic an easy task. Apart from the above mentioned list, graters, peeler, measuring cups, spoons and strainers come in very handy while fixing a quick meal.

Another important kitchen equipment that every vegan should possess is a blender and a food processor. In order to get your healthy juices and delicious smoothies ready in a jiffy, a good quality blender works like a charm. All you need to do is put all your ingredients and blend your way to good health. A food processor is also a very useful appliance as it makes chopping and grinding very easy and causes less hassle. When you are in a hurry, you can drop them in and have your ingredients ready to continue your cooking spree. It is also great for making desserts, especially cakes, pastries and doughnuts, the vegan style of course!

If you have some extra bucks to shell, then a dedicated juicer is a good option as you can save it to process your juices alone. The blender can be used for all ingredients but the residual essence of it might tamper with your juices and the taste might be affected. A juicer ensures that your juices are brimming with its individual essence and absolutely delicious.

If you are more of a quick fixer and prefer cooking methods that require less time, then owning a pressure cooker is a must. It will soften your vegetables in a few seconds and have them imbibe the flavor very well. It takes less time and eases the cooking process. These are some of the basic equipments that you require in order to set up a vegan kitchen.

Chapter 5 - Vegan Juices and Smoothies Recipes

This serves as an ideal option for all those who have hectic mornings getting chores done and rushing off for work. All you need to do is throw some ingredients, blend and you are done. Smoothies and juices are certainly healthy options that can be taken any time of the day. It is delicious, filling and very healthy. It keeps you going steady with a happy belly even post lunchtime. Read on for some interesting recipes that guarantee taste and extreme energy.

Green Energy Smoothie

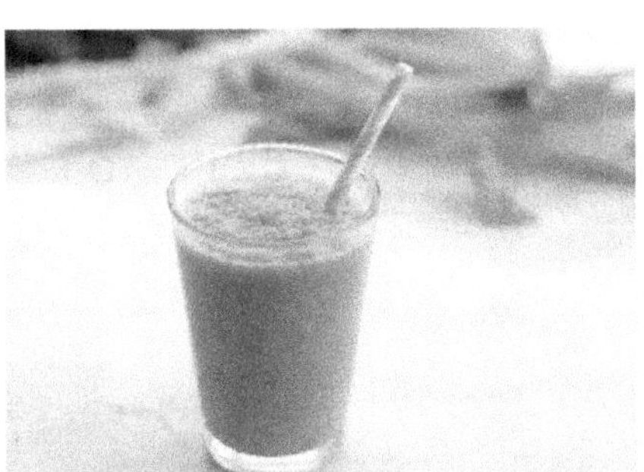

It is an absolute treat to your taste buds, as well as your eyes as it looks just gorgeous. The green shade is very inviting and a glass full of this goodness will instantly boost your energy levels and keep you feeling active and strong. It is also a great option for all those on a weight loss spree. It also makes use of green tea, which has been known for its detox and weight loss characteristics.

Servings: 2

Ingredients:

- 3 cups spinach (raw)
- 2 cups melon (cubed)
- 1 cucumber (seeded and chopped)
- 1 cup green tea (organic)
- 1 tsp lemon juice
- ½ inch ginger root (fresh)

Method

- Transfer all the ingredients to a blender.

- Blend it well till it reaches a smooth consistency.
- Transfer the contents to a serving glass and enjoy.

Apple Pie Smoothie

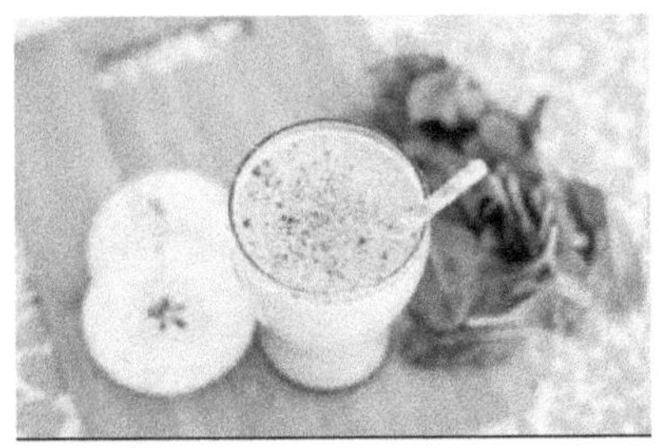

This recipe is a must try for all the health conscious individuals out there. It serves as a great post workout option and fills your belly without sensing the need to grab breakfast. It is high in protein and carbohydrates. The walnuts used provide a good dose of the healthy fat that one requires to feel active and strong all day long. Try and sip it for a great start to your day.

Servings: 2

Ingredients

- ½ cup water
- 1tsp walnuts
- ½ tsp cinnamon (freshly grounded)
- ½ cup apple juice (unsweetened)
- ¼ tsp maple syrup
- 1 cucumber
- 1 apple (chopped)
- 2 cups spinach
- ¼ avocado (chopped)
- 5 ice cubes
- A pinch of nutmeg (grounded)

Method

● In a blender, add all the ingredients.

● Blend for a few seconds till it reaches the desired consistency. Repeat if you need it to be smoother and lump free.

● Relish it while it's still cold and delicious.

Healthy Tomato Juice

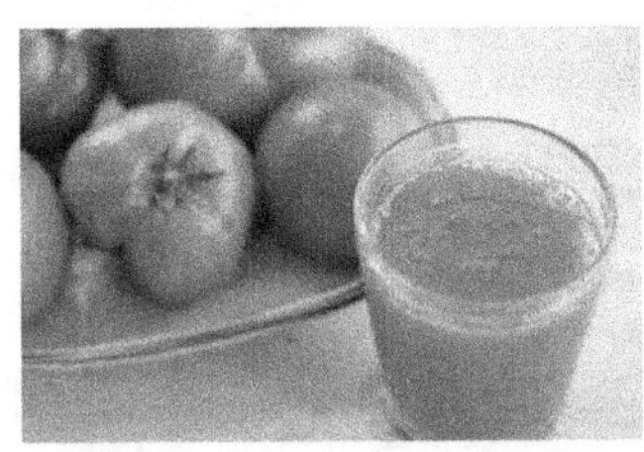

Tomatoes serve as an excellent option for all those who like a tinge of tanginess to their drink. Besides looking red and extremely beautiful, tomatoes are rich in potassium, vitamins A and C. They are low in sodium, cholesterol and calories. It serves as a great form of blood purifier and also has anti-oxidant properties. It prevents muscular degeneration and improves eyesight and skin. It also promotes extra energy when coupled with a healthy breakfast.

Servings: 2

Ingredients

- 3 cups tomatoes (chopped)
- 1 stalk celery
- 1 cucumber
- ½ tsp sea salt
- 2pinches of pepper

Method

- Take a blender and add the tomatoes, cucumber and celery and blend it to a smooth consistency.
- Season it with salt and pepper.

High Energy Juice

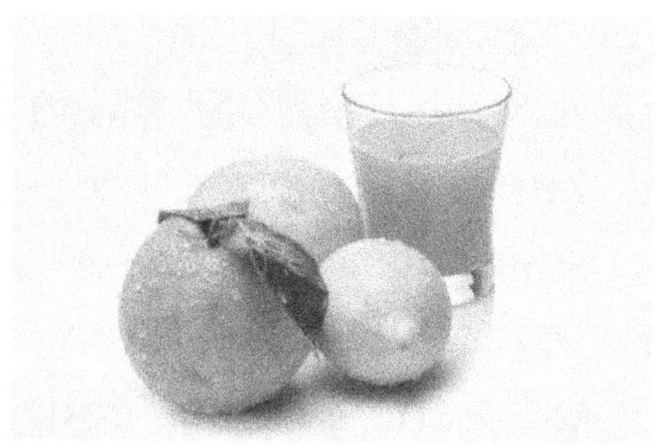

The name explains it all. Yes, it is a drink that makes you feel refreshed, energetic and of course happy. It comes with the goodness of carrots and mint, among several other ingredients. Carrots are great for the eyes and help to develop better eyesight. Have it early in the morning and you will feel your best throughout the day.

Servings: 2

Ingredients

- 4 carrots (chopped)
- 1 orange (peeled)
- ½ lemon (peeled)
- 3 mint leaves
- ¼ inch ginger root (fresh)

Method

- Wash and thoroughly clean all the ingredients.
- Add it to a blender and blend till it is lump free and reaches the desired consistency.

Chapter 6 - Vegan Breakfast Recipes

Breakfast is undoubtedly the most important meal of the day as it fuels your body up after many hours of fasting all through the night. In order to kick start your day on a good note, it is important to plan and consume healthy and smart breakfast options. It is necessary as it gets your metabolism running which in turns leads to more burning of calories throughout the day. It will also prevent you from binge eating later throughout the day and will also keep your energy levels going high and strong. Read on for more vegan breakfast ideas.

Quinoa Cakes

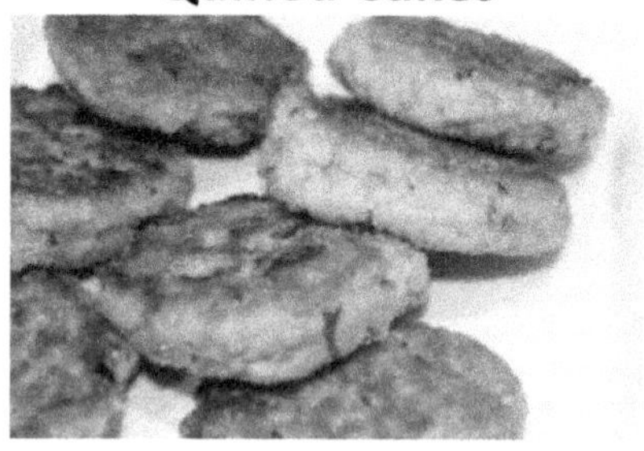

Who doesn't love cakes? Yes, we all adore them! The good news is that this recipe calls for a healthy cake which you can gorge on endlessly without feeling guilty about your weight. It uses quinoa which is an excellent ingredient for promoting good health and fitness. It makes a filling meal and still keeps a tab on your weight. Quinoa is rich in protein, fiber, minerals, iron and magnesium among other beneficial factors. This super grain is known to enhance the metabolism and promotes energy production in the cells. It also helps to reduce diabetes, blood pressure and several other ailments.

Servings: 3

Ingredients

- 1 1/2 cups quinoa (cooked)
- 2 tbsp ground flax
- 6 tbsp water
- 1 cup kale (chopped)
- 1/2 cup rolled oats (grounded into smooth powder)
- 1/2 cup sweet potato(grated)

- 1/4 cup sun-dried tomatoes (chopped)
- 1/4 cup sunflower seeds
- 1/4 cup basil leaves (chopped)
- 2 tbsp onion (finely diced)
- 1 clove garlic (minced)
- 1 tbsp runny tahini paste
- 1 1/2 tbsp dried oregano
- 1 1/2 tbsp red or white vinegar
- 3 tbsp all-purpose flour (gluten-free)
- Salt and red pepper flakes to taste

Method

- Let's begin by preheating the oven to 400F.
- Grease a baking tray and line it with butter paper and set aside.
- Mix water and the ground flax in a small bowl and set it aside for few minutes till it thickens.
- Now take a large bowl and add all the ingredients. Mix well.
- Include the ground flax, water mixture and mix well till all the ingredients are well-blended and incorporated.

• Dampen your palms and take a little ball of the prepared dough and make it into the shape of small patties.
• Space it out evenly and place them on the baking tray.
• Push it into the oven and bake for about 15 minutes on one side. Flip them and continue for another 10 minutes.
• When both the sides are golden brown and crisp, it is time to remove them from the oven.
• Allow it to cool and then enjoy your savory healthy cake to your heart's content.

Oatmeal Squares

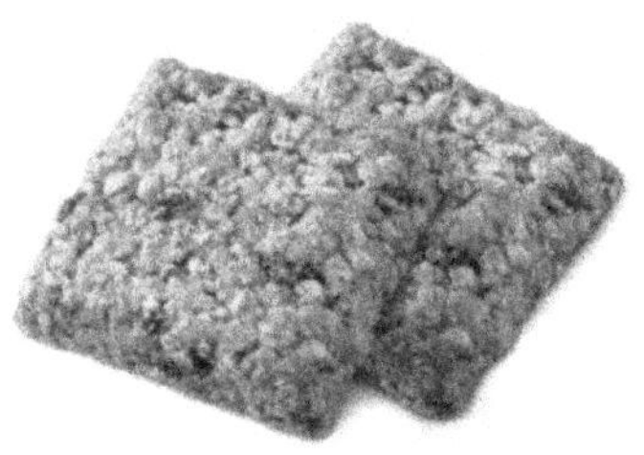

Oats qualify as a healthy and filling breakfast ingredient. It starts your day on a good and satiated note and you don't feel the need to snack until much later. It also prevents you from over eating or binge eating as a small quantity of oats is enough to serve the purpose. Oats are known as whole grains and they work wonders in reducing risk of diabetes, blood pressure and cholesterol. They also eliminate risks of coronary artery diseases, colorectal cancer and several other ailments. They are rich in fiber and umpteen minerals that provide the body with all the essentials that it requires.

Servings: 2

Ingredients

- 1 tbsp ground flax
- 3 tbsp water
- 1/2 cup pumpkin purée (unsweetened)
- 3/4 cup coconut sugar
- 1 tsp vanilla extract
- 1/2 tsp baking soda
- 1/2 tsp sea salt
- 1 1/2 tsp cinnamon (grounded)
- 1/2 tsp ginger(grounded)
- 1/8 tsp nutmeg (grounded)
- 3/4 cup oats flour
- 3/4 cup oats (rolled)
- 3/4 cup almond flour
- 1 tsp arrowroot powder
- 1/2 cup pecan halves (chopped)
- 2 tbsp non-dairy chocolate chips

Method

• Preheat the oven to 350F. Grease and line a baking tray.

• Mix water and ground flax and set aside to thicken.

- Take a large mixing bowl and add pumpkin puree and sugar and blend it until well-incorporated.
- Pour the vanilla extract over the flax mixture. Mix well.
- Include the salt, baking soda, cinnamon, nutmeg and ginger and mix till everything is well combined.
- Add the remaining ingredients and fold well so that it takes the shape of sticky dough.
- Place the dough on the tray and level it. Throw in some chocolate chip cookies and push it into the oven.
- Bake for about 15 - 20 minutes till golden brown.
- Cut into squares and enjoy.

Quick No Bake Protein Bar

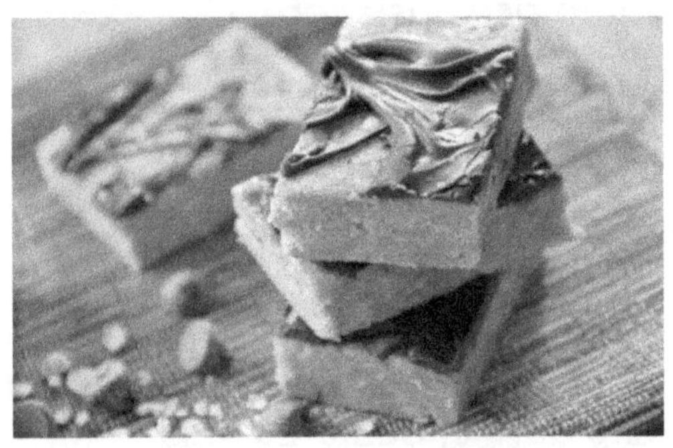

Getting your daily dose of proteins is an absolutely must and this recipe is surely a change from the usual protein rich based meals. The best part about this recipe is that it is very easy to put together and requires less time. Grab a few bars before you head out and you will surely feel satisfied and strong for a good number of hours. Try it and be amazed.

Servings: 3

Ingredients

- 1.5 cups rolled oats (blended into a flour)

- 1/2 cup vegan protein powder (unsweetened)
- 1/2 cup rice crisp cereal
- 1/2 tsp sea salt
- 1/2 cup peanut butter or almond butter
- 1/2 cup maple syrup
- 1 tsp vanilla extract
- 3 tbsp dark chocolate chips
- 1/2 tbsp coconut oil

Method

- Take a tray or a square pan and line it with parchment paper.
- In a large bowl, add the oats flour, protein powder, rice crisp and salt and mix well.
- In another bowl, combine the wet ingredients: butter, maple syrup and the vanilla extract and mix well.
- Mix the dry ingredients with the wet ingredients. Stir properly to make sure everything is well combined.

- Add it to the earlier prepared tray and roll it out with a pastry roller.
- Keep it in the freezer for over ten minutes.
- In a pan, add the chocolate chips and the coconut oil and melt it over a low flame till it reaches a smooth consistency.
- Once set, remove the bars, and pour the melted mixture over it and pop it again into the freezer.
- Remove it, cut it into bars and enjoy.
- You can save it for one whole week provided it is sealed shut in an air tight container and rested in the freezer.

Chapter 7 - Vegan Side Dishes

When the regular meals become a routine, it is nice to deviate and spice up the table with some interesting side dishes. They can be enjoyed along with the main dish or even as appetizers and helps exercise your taste buds a great deal. Try out these simple and delicious recipes and you will crave for more!

Zucchini and Corn Combo

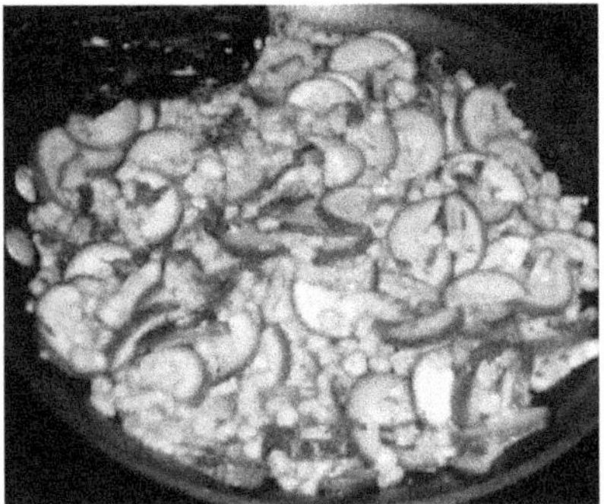

This is an interesting mix which tastes amazing and also provides umpteen health benefits. Zucchini is rich in dietary fibers and helps to eliminate risks of colon cancers and also cures complaints of constipation. It contains no content of fats or cholesterol and thereby makes for a healthy meal option.

Servings: 6

Ingredients

- 1/4 cup vegetable broth
- 1 ½ cups onion (chopped)
- 3 medium zucchini (sliced)
- 1 package frozen corn (organic)
- 1 tsp dried oregano
- Salt to taste
- Black pepper to taste
- 5 cups plum tomatoes(chopped)

Method

• To a pan, add the vegetable broth and heat it over a medium flame.

• Add the onions and cook in the broth till tender. Stir continuously to avoid it from sticking to the pan.

• Adjust broth or water accordingly

• Add the zucchini. Cook for a couple of minutes, while stirring frequently.

- Now add the remaining ingredients and bring the mixture to a boil.
- Let it simmer for about 20 to 25 minutes over low flame till the zucchini is cooked and tender.
- Transfer it to a serving dish and relish while it's still hot and delicious.

Seasoned Potato salad

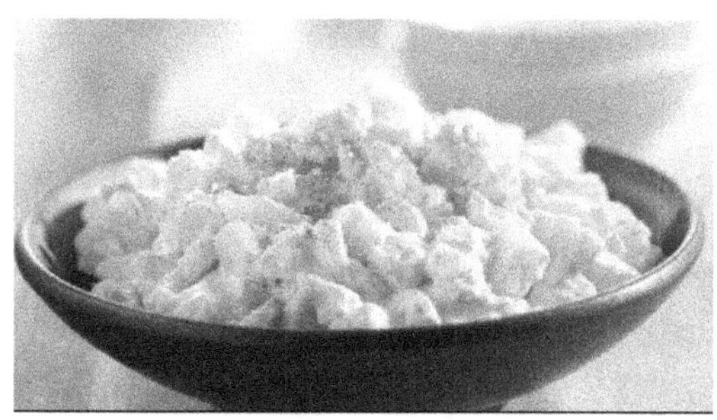

Salads are great as a side dish because they can be experimented till it matches the chef's fancy. Throw in several ingredients of your choice and a healthy platter is all ready to be relished. Try this potato salad for your dose of carbohydrates to keep you going strong. It titillates your taste buds without adding to the weight.

Servings: 5

Ingredients

- 5 <u>potatoes</u>, (unpeeled and cubed)
- 2 <u>carrots</u> (shredded)
- 1 stalk celery (diced)
- 4 onions,(diced)
- 1 cup vegan mayonnaise
- 2 Tbsp organic soy sauce
- 1 tsp basil
- 1 tsp paprika
- 1 tsp garlic powder
- 1 tsp oregano
- Sea salt and black pepper to taste

Method

• Take a pan and fill it with water. Add salt. Add the cubed potatoes and cook it till they are slightly tender but firm.

• Take care not to overcook it.

• Drain and set it aside to cool.

● Take a large mixing bowl, add the remaining ingredients, the potatoes and top it off with the seasonings. Combine it well.

● Serve it chilled for the extra zing.

Chapter 8 - Vegan Main Dishes

Now that we have tackled the breakfast and the side dish options, let's move on to some main course dishes which can be served for lunch as well as dinner. Most of these recipes are easy to fix and very healthy. A good serving of it will be sufficient to keep our tummy feeling happy, healthy and strong. Keep reading!

Vegetable stir fry

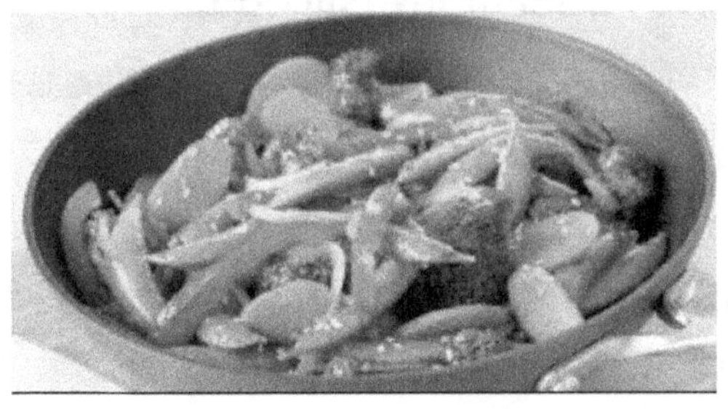

It serves as a mouthwatering dish which combines the goodness of vegetables and is topped with an interesting seasoning. Vegetables are essential for providing your body with its daily essentials. You can experiment and add as many vegetables as you prefer based on your preference and taste. It is surely a must try!

Servings: 7

Ingredients

- ¼ cup canola oil
- 2 carrots (chopped)
- 1 cup potatoes (chopped)
- 1 cup lotus root (peeled and sliced)
- ¼ cup maple syrup
- ¼ cup soy sauce
- 1 tsp sesame oil
- 1tbsp sesame seeds (toasted)
- 2 scallions (sliced finely)

Method

- Begin by preheating the oven to 375F.
- Heat the canola oil in a pan and add the carrots and potatoes to it.
- Cook it over medium heat till they are golden brown.
- Transfer it to a tray and push it into the oven. Allow it to roast for about 20 minutes till the vegetables are cooked and tender.

- Remove from pan and add the content to the pan over medium flame,
- Include the lotus roots, maple syrup and soy sauce and cook it over low heat, while stirring continuously.
- Cook for another ten minutes till the mixture thicken and takes the consistency of syrup.
- Cook the vegetables till they are well coated with this syrupy mixture.
- Finally, throw in the sesame oil, sesame seeds and scallions to the pan.
- Serve immediately for better results.

Vegan Pasta with Broccoli

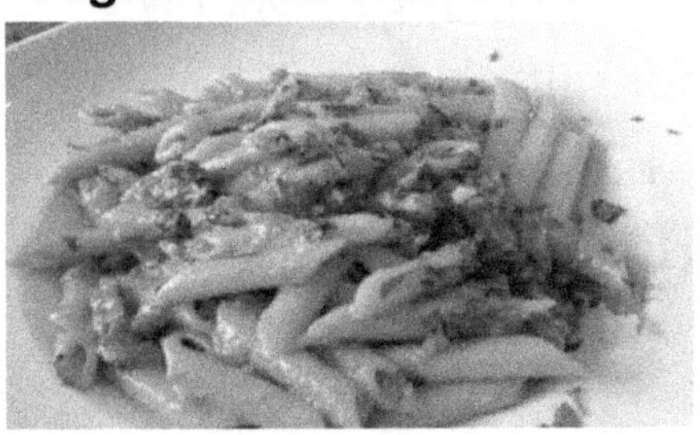

When we crave Italian, most of us tend to choose pasta over other dishes and rightly so. It is delicious, filling and so easy to prepare. If you are a fellow pasta lover, then this recipe is certainly a keeper. It is combined with the goodness of broccoli, which is a very effective anti-oxidant. It is also useful for preventing cancer, reducing allergies and inflammation, keeps cholesterol in check and promotes overall bones and heart health.

Servings: 5

Ingredients

- 4 tbsp extra virgin olive oil
- 1 head broccoli (cut into inches)
- 8 cloves garlic (thinly sliced)
- 1 tsp dried oregano
- 1/2 tsp red chili flakes
- 1 can of tomatoes (roughly chopped)
- Kosher salt
- 500 grams penne pasta
- 1/4 cup parsley leaves (chopped)

Method

• Take a large pan and add oil to it. Allow it to simmer on a low flame.

• Throw in the chopped broccoli and cook till it is lightly brown in color.

• Add the garlic, oregano and chilli flakes and sauté.

• Stir constantly to prevent it from burning.

• Include the tomatoes and allow the mixture to boil, once done, reduce and allow it to simmer till the broccoli is tender.

• Season it with salt.

• Take a large container and add water and salt to it and keep it on a high flame. Once the water begins to boil, add the pasta and cook till it is 'al Dante' to the point. Drain and set aside.

• Once the mixture is ready, add the cooked pasta and mix well.

• Garnish with parsley leaves, olive oil and serve hot.

Chapter 9 - Vegan Desserts

After a hearty meal that consists of appetizers, side dishes and main course, all one can dream of are desserts, to bring the meal to a satisfying and sweet end. When your sweet tooth just refuses to obey your commands, head over to the kitchen and fix these easy vegan desserts and all will be well. Surprise your family to a sweet treat that is healthy yet fulfilling.

Banana Bread Muffin Tops

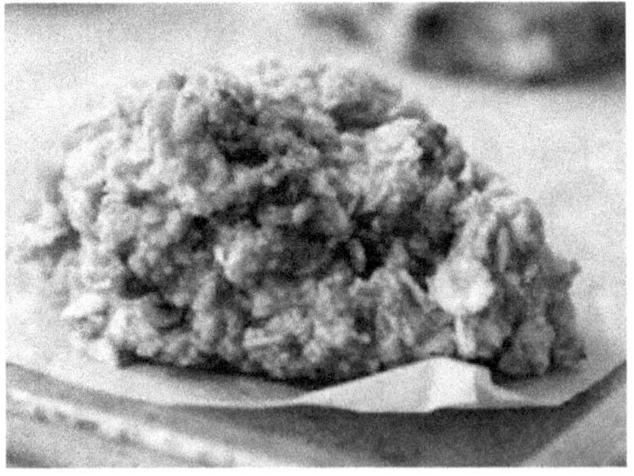

It is certainly a treat to die for! Muffins are delicious and one just cannot stop till the entire tray is licked clean. To top the muffin goodness with bananas and dates, it surely takes it to another level altogether. Try it and this will instantly become your favorite dessert option of all times.

Servings: 3

Ingredients

- 2 large ripe bananas (peeled)
- 1/2 cup dates (pitted)
- 1/4 cup virgin coconut oil
- 1 tsp vanilla extract
- 1 tsp cinnamon
- 1 tsp baking powder
- 1/4 + 1/8 tsp sea salt
- 2 cups rolled oats (rolled and divided)
- 3-4 tbsp chocolate chips(nondairy)

Method

● Preheat the oven to around 350F and grease the baking tray. Set it aside.

● To a food processor or a blender, add the bananas, dates, coconut oil and vanilla extract/ process until smooth.

- Include the cinnamon, baking powder and salt and run it once again through the processor.
- Add half of the oats and process the mixture for a few seconds and turn it off. The oats should not be fine, just course will be sufficient.
- Transfer the contents to another bowl. Add the remaining oats and chocolate chips and fold it well into the mixture.
- Take a spoonful of the dough and place it on the lined tray.
- Bake for about ten minutes, change the position of the tray and continue baking for another ten minutes.
- Allow it to cool and dig into the heavenly goodness.

Coffee Cookies

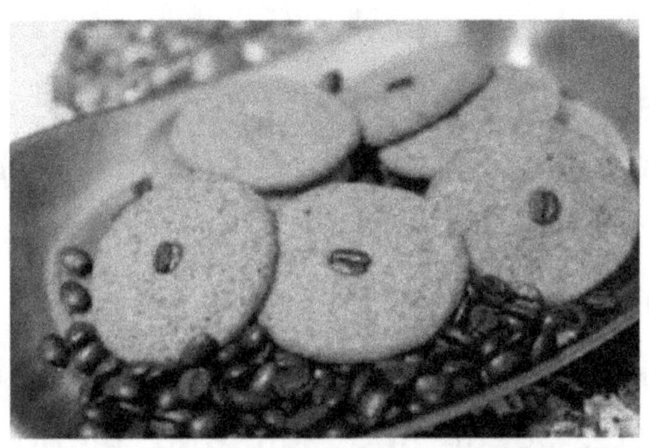

Cookies certainly classify as comfort food, which not only helps you to unwind and de-stress after a long and tiring day, but also leaves you feeling joyous ad satisfied. This interesting combination of coffee and walnuts is surely a must try. The best part is that it is so easy to make and can be ready in a jiffy.

Servings: 5

Ingredients

- 1 cup all-purpose flour
- 1/2 cup walnut (chopped)

- 6 tbsp raw cane sugar

1/8 tsp salt

1 tsp freshly ground coffee beans

3/4 tsp vanilla extract

1 cup butter (unsalted/cut into cubes)

Method

- Take a food processor and add, flour, walnuts, sugar and salt and blend until smooth.
- Add the ground coffee beans and blend once again.
- Add the butter and vanilla essence and adjust the consistency with a little water.
- Place the dough balls on the tray and freeze it for about 2 to 3 hours.
- Remove it from the fridge and bake in a preheated oven for about 15 minutes at 350F.
- Bake till it is golden brown, cool and serve.

Chapter 10 – Conclusion

This complete guide provides all information that one requires to live life the vegan way. The recipes are easy to make and serve the purpose of a healthy diet plan. It provides all the basic requirements of the body and adheres to all needs in terms of vitamins and minerals. If you are new to this arena, then this guide will surely guide and assist you in making the right choices. If you are facing some medical complication, it is best advised to consult your doctor before you make any changes in your diet and lifestyle. A vegan lifestyle can be easily practiced by anyone, irrespective of the gender, age, size or preferences. Go ahead and live life the healthy and energetic way. Go vegan!

About the Author

Luis Crump is author of several cookbooks on Vegan diet. He has written research papers on the topic and currently lives in California.

www.ingramcontent.com/pod-product-compliance
Lightning Source LLC
Chambersburg PA
CBHW060952050726
47592CB00003B/1204